DARE TO BE HAPPIER

AN INTRODUCTION TO THE MAGIC OF JOURNALING TO TRANSFORM YOUR LIFE

CAROLINE JOHNSTONE

"Stop looking for happiness in the place where you lost it"

CONTENTS

This edition first published in 2018 by Snowdrop Press
Unit 1
13 Pennylands View
Auchinleck
Ayrshire
KA18 2LG
www.daretobehappier.com

A catalogue record for this book is available from the British Library
ISBN 978-0-9561922-1-9
10 9 8 7 6 5 4 3 2 1/13 14 15 16

Contact the author directly by email:
caroline@daretobehappier.com

INTRODUCTION

I dare people to be happier. I help people figure out what is keeping them stuck, making them unhappy or fearful, and then support and empower them to make the changes they want to live the life they really want. We like our comfort zones so much that this can often be less than totally easy to do – even though we know we want to – and that's why I know it needs courage. I also know that anyone's courage is lying in wait for action. As Mark Twain said, "Courage is resistance to fear, mastery of fear, not absence of fear." It's doing something different, regardless of how you feel about it. You can't rely on these feelings to guide you as they won't let you move. As Susan Jeffers said, you've got to feel the fear – and do it anyway.

I dare others to be happier because I've been

deeply unhappy in the past myself, but changed my life. I've been so unhappy that I have felt terribly stuck, unable to see any options to change things, and that led to me losing the ability to feel anything deeply as I numbed myself, and so I lost hope of a better life. Over the years, I have learned that my thinking was at fault – as that then led to how I felt and how I acted, or didn't act. I've also learned a huge number of tools and techniques that make sure I am happier and stay that way much more often, and I now consciously create my reality and a better life. The main tool I use personally and in my courses and coaching is journaling, because I came to realise that the answers are already there, if I just allow myself to access them. We all have a deep inner wisdom, a knowing, that would guide us if we stopped listening to other people's desires and plans for our lives and stopped over-riding what it's guiding us to do. We owe it to ourselves and the world to step into our power, open our heart to this wisdom and live lives we love. This joy of living is contagious - the happier you are, the happier others will be too (and if they aren't, that is their responsibility).

OUR THINKING CREATES OUR REALITY

The same is of course true for unhappiness – and

therefore both are like viruses that can spread like any pandemic panic can. When it's high profile suicides – and with the impact of social media in spreading stories – then this really becomes worrying, and can lead to trends of copycat acts. Following such stories, there's often a flurry of experts warning that these may trigger further suicides (this is known as suicide contagion) in people who had already been considering it, but now have much more focus on this step as an option because it's in the news and seems to be "everywhere." It's even got a name- the "Werther effect," after a book written in 1774 by Goethe. This was a story of unrequited love and a black and white idealism that meant the main character could only see an empty life, and so he committed suicide. It was the thinking that led to the act, but what happened was that others who were thinking the same way did the same thing. It's a perfect example of how thinking creates reality – and it doesn't have to be like that.

A HAPPINESS VIRUS

In 2009, I started to really think about how easily groups and individuals could quickly be affected by outside issues. A pandemic was forecast, and some people really did get sick, but the media blew this up to be something that was much more serious than it ever was, and created a panic about it that baffled me. An article by Simon Jenkins in The Guardian in May 2009* summed up exactly how I felt, including his comments on who benefitted from such panic (which wasn't you or me, and it wasn't the businesses that went bust as a result).

Since it was the thinking that was creating the panic about something negative, I started to wonder what would happen if something positive swept the world instead, as an antidote? That question led to the launch of my Facebook page Happiness Virus. I knew all about positive psychology and how our thinking controls our lives – that what we focus on, we see more of, and that we create our reality from what we think, feel and do. If the life we lead starts with our thinking, how could I encourage people to see life differently?

This really mattered to me for living my purpose – but it also really mattered to me very personally as I'd learned how vital this was to enable me to deal with high level anxiety and depression so I could live my best life - and I had two student daughters who for different reasons were both feeling pretty down around this time. I knew they'd want to help their mum, so I asked them go away and find me articles, photos and quotes that I could post about how your thinking or actions improves or changes lives, the power of gratitude, what to do if you were feeling stuck, how to be happier. Full confession – which they both now know – is that I did this with the full intention of changing their perspective.

And it worked. It changed their lives. Now, they both work (as you do need to work – it's part of that daring mindset) at finding positives, gifts in the bad times or in reframing how we looked back at these, at doing what supports and nurtures them to live happier lives. My youngest daughter Jenni has a great life full of travel and adventures as she runs her own business as a mortgage consultant while training to be a pension consultant. My eldest daughter Emma is now the Head of Positive Education for a group of schools in Dubai where children, parents and teachers are taught how to look after their own wellbeing by developing growth mindsets, and understanding what makes them happy. In March 2018 they all enjoyed a visit from Meik Wiking, CEO of The Happiness Research Institute and author of The Little Books of Hygge and Lykke, who loved what he saw happening there.

DARE TO BE HAPPY?

In time, I changed the Facebook group to Dare To Be Happy because I'd come to realise that people often need encouragement to make changes, even tiny changes – but that was what was ultimately what was needed to improve their life. I knew myself how hard it could be to feel fear and act, how often fear would keep me paralysed where I was. I also knew that I was mainly responsible for my own happiness, an inside job, so if I wanted to be happy, I had to act; there was no magic solution. I made a lot of changes to my life that improved it hugely, but soon realised that a relentless determination to pursue happiness doesn't make you happy. A similar determination to get up and just be happy every day, all day long isn't realistic (though you can choose to make those choices moment by moment).

Truth was, I came to see that I'd be living a lie – and encouraging others to do the same- by saying just be happy. It just isn't always possible. If you are going through major illness, grief or life changes due to external circumstances or your own fair hand, you aren't being real if you insist on permanent happiness. There are times in life when you simply need to nurture yourself and be gentle, and critically, to allow yourself to feel the reality of all of your emotions, not numb them or ignore them – but even in those times, it is possible to dare to be happier. I changed my page name again, and knew this was what I wanted to teach; the same thing I needed to learn. There's no-one on the earth who can't dare to be a bit happier than they are now. At very difficult times, this might mean that you switch your phone off, stop using social media, or decide to take a first step to look after yourself well again, towards a new normal life, or get up and get dressed at a "normal" time.

GETTING UNSTUCK AND FINDING A NEW NORMAL

What I've found through my research, my coaching, conversations with hundreds of people going through such times, is that what is really important is that you stop yourself getting stuck in a place where you allow your life to simply stop, where you get afraid to try again, live again, love again. You don't want to be stuck, and you don't need to be stuck. I have met so many people who have lived through life changing diagnoses and still managed to dare to be happier. Others may have attempted suicide, experienced crippling anxiety or depression and fear its return, have left violent or abusive relationships, lost children to illness or accidents, partners to violent crime, been made redundant from a job they loved – but their lives have turned around because they too dared to be happier. They are living meaningful lives, where they have found ways to get up most mornings, use their pain to create lasting change for others, found peace with their new normal. That's when living really takes courage - to determine you will redefine what a good life looks like *and* live it.

DARE TO BE HAPPIER

You need to dare to be happier: I need to too. You won't often just think or talk yourself into transformation. That's why campaigns focussing on talking about better mental health are limiting, because you could talk about how you are thinking or feeling until the cows come home – but until you make some changes in both of these areas, and until you act, nothing will change. Medication will only numb or reduce symptoms – and remember that big pharmaceutical companies have no interest in curing people if that would affect their profits. In 2017, the World Health Organisation said that depression was "the leading cause of ill health and disability worldwide" and that there had been an 18% increase in this area alone in the ten years between 2005 and 2015. How can this be, when our lives are so much easier in so many ways than they were for our grandparents or great grandparents?

The issues are multi-factorial, but scientific evidence shows that materialism doesn't make us happier (we need some money, but it's not all about the money and can't be because of hedonistic adaptation), that our fascination with celebrity and the perfectionism shown on social media impacts us. Our loss of communities, our failure to exercise, to get into nature enough, our key relationships or lack of them (created in person, not online), our environment, our sense of purpose (not living an empty life but doing something for others), our background and our genetics are just some of what impacts our happiness and wellbeing. There are many different definitions of wellbeing from country or council/area definitions to those by organisations like The World Health Organisation or The National Office of Statistics. Perhaps Ereaut and Whiting (2008) summarise it best when they say it's "what a group or groups of people collectively agree makes a good life."

THE MAGICAL INGREDIENT FOR YOUR BEST LIFE

And that's where journaling comes in; it's the magical ingredient for living your best life – and scientific research confirms this to be the case. It's not magical in the sense of any sort of supernatural or mysterious force from the outside being involved, but for the transformation it can effect from the inside. It allows us to tap into our own inner wisdom, change how we think - and change how we see our world (and the wider world in general).

We describe things as magical when the seemingly impossible happens, special powers are displayed, or when amazing results appear. The Oxford English Dictionary says that something can be described as magical when it is very effective in producing the desired results, like some sort of magical ingredient.

When we regularly journal, we start to realise that many of the beliefs, values, attitudes that we've held to date (and stories we've held on to) are no longer serving us. Journaling changes our destiny, so we are no longer a victim of our past but in control of our future, for in accessing our inner wisdom, we also learn to listen to our past and see it differently, and then let it go so we have room to make the changes a better future requires.

That might mean that we look after ourselves better, set firmer boundaries, become aware of our inner critic and manage it, or improve our relationships or living environments. It may mean that we go for that promotion or change jobs entirely, tap into our creativity, become more present, make healthier choices. Or we may do something else entirely that improves our happiness and wellbeing. Ultimately, the magic of journaling is not just in what we write, but in what we do as a result. Your life right now is the one you've created. That's a fact, however unpleasant that thought may be. The choices you've made, based on how you've been thinking, led to how you responded to what life brought you – and don't beat yourself up about this.

Even when your past has been less than totally positive (or worse), it is how you responded to that – your thoughts and actions – that brought you to this point. What you did and what you failed to do – your successes, failures and mistakes, your actions and inactions happened when you were doing the best you could with the tools you had based on your experience and background at that point. And this point – where you are now- is the point of possibility.

THE MAGIC OF JOURNALING LIES IN ITS POWER TO TRANSFORM

For that was then; this is now - and the good news is that journaling will transform both your present *and* your future. In fact, journaling helps create change so much more easily than you could imagine right now.

It is a discipline that creates a space for you to invest in yourself. When your life's too busy, doing some things that matter and many that don't, or when it's mainly concentrated on the needs of others timetables or demands, you don't realise that YOU are last on your To Do List. When was the last time you slowed down enough to think, breathe, recharge your batteries, process your emotions or observe your life?

Journaling creates a safe place to explore your world, discover patterns that are less than totally helpful because they mean you sabotage success, see what really isn't working, identify the elements of your life you want to change, and then enable you to start to make plans and take action to make these happen.

I have always written diaries and journals of some sort, and when my life got out of kilter or when I made my biggest mistakes, it would always be because I wasn't spending any time journaling. I would be unable to see options. I would forget to listen to my heart. I would look for answers in the wrong places. Had I given myself the time to reflect on my life or the choices I might make, I could and would have made many conscious changes.

Examining your life on a regular basis (your thoughts, hopes and fears, actions, choices, values, beliefs and attitudes), connects you to your heart and inner wisdom. In my younger life, I had been in very dark places where I saw no options; journaling helped me see that I always had more options than I believed. In 2002, I read Cheryl Richardson's book Stand Up For Your Life, a book that encouraged you to write down answers to guided questions, and it changed my life, sending me on a quest to really explore journaling. That's when I started to see how powerful it was when used as a regular practice.

I try to journal every day. If I don't set time aside first thing, it doesn't always happen, as "life" gets in the way, though even then you might find me scribbling something in another notebook on the train journey home, or before I go to sleep. I've found that without fail, when I do start my day by journaling, I have a better day. I set intentions for how I want my day to go, perhaps spend some time reviewing the day before, ask myself questions about what's on my mind at that point, or use one of the many journaling tools available.

FIND THE MAGIC

It's almost time to dive in to the learning. In the first part of the book we will look at the history of journaling as a tool or practice, the "rules" of journaling, why journaling matters, the science around therapeutic journaling. In the second part, we look at seven of the key tools you can use. The final part of the book gives you guided questions to use for each week – a year to really think about your life and what you want from it.

If you've never journaled before, then start small. Set yourself up for success. Don't decide you will now write every day if you know you have a habit of failing to keep your promises to yourself. (Learn to change that habit anyway, so you can promise yourself that you will live your best life, and invest in practices that support this, for that's a promise worth keeping). Carve out some time by getting up earlier, watching one less TV programme or by spending less time surfing the net or on social media when you wake up.

If you don't have time to invest 15 or 20 minutes in yourself, then you are too busy. Since journaling will help you see why that is and how to change it, you can't lose by this time investment! Start by setting a timer you don't end up running late if you've limited time or buses to catch. Just start writing, and see what "comes up." Or ask yourself a question about the biggest thing that is bothering you (like *why* is it bothering you, or what options do you have). Or buy a journal on a particular theme that has a number of questions for you to work your way through. It doesn't matter what you do to start, it just matters that you start.

For in starting, you will find your old dreams and dust them off or create new dreams. You will reconnect with who you really are and what matters to you. You will find the courage to take the risk of going after what you want to follow your own path and live the life you want.

You will learn to slow your life down and pay attention to it, listening and losing your must do lists, learning to be present, and to practice self-care. You will find it easier to choose a lighter way of being, start seeing different results by changing thoughts, beliefs and actions, and find that you are wiser in looking after your own happiness and wellbeing.

And if that isn't magic, I don't know what is.

https://www.theguardian.com/commentis-free/2009/may/05/swine-flu-panic

TO LOVE MEANS TO LISTEN

To love means to listen. Listening is a very important practice.
There is a voice calling us, and it wants us to listen.
It may be that our body is calling us and wants us to listen to
our body.
It may be our feelings that are calling us and want us to listen
to them.
It may be our perceptions are calling us and want us to listen.
It is very important for us to pay attention to the voice.
The capacity of listening to ourselves is the foundation of the
capacity of listening to others.
The capacity to love others depends on the capacity of loving
ourselves.

— THICH NHAT HANH

I

AN INTRODUCTION TO THE MAGIC OF JOURNALING TO TRANSFORM YOUR LIFE

1. A BRIEF HISTORY OF JOURNALLING

A JOURNAL IS NOT A DIARY

The word "journaling" is often used for what in practice is meant by simply keeping a diary that is a record of each day or week - but it's much more than that. Throughout the centuries, people have used diaries to record daily life and world events. We see this in ancient cave paintings and hieroglyphics, modern day tree carvings and graffiti, and in the diaries where people have recorded events, lives and thinking for posterity, hoping to live on in what they have written.

For that reason, diaries can be a fascinating glimpse of life, becoming a living history in retrospect, recording memories which range from the mundane - I know of a man who simply records the daily weather and gardening activities - to the extraordinary. The diary written by Samuel Pepys gives us a fascinating record of his personal life, 17th Century daily life and significant events like war and the Great Plague and Fires of London. Travel journals record real journeys, adventures, or reflections on these by the individuals concerned, or by others interested in the journey. For instance, NASA has studied the effects of isolation and confinement in space travel by reviewing the journals of astronauts (concluding that future astronauts need training in handling conflict, cultural differences, coping strategies and communication!).

Where a journal differs from a diary is the insight it gives the writer into their *own* life, as it is being written, or in reviewing what has been written. With the benefit of hindsight, Anne Frank's Diary gives us a poignant insight into the horror of life for Jews in Germany during the Second World War.

At the outset she probably didn't know that was what she would end up doing, but that changed, and she wanted to record what was happening. Yet, she found that she also needed to write about the experience of being a young woman growing up in hiding.

As we read her diary, we almost feel we know her, because she shares some of the same thoughts and feelings we had about growing up (while sharing other thoughts and feelings we could never imagine). We can't, however, know her fully through her diaries, because in a place where there was no real privacy, where she would write always knowing someone *may* try to read it, only the bravest would write wholly from the heart – a commitment we make when we decide to take journaling seriously. We need privacy to be wholeheartedly honest, or to find ways of writing with total honesty without fear of judgement or intrusion.

CONNECTING TO YOUR INNER WISDOM

Journals always include a combination of reflection, deep honesty and journeying; when you journal, you're not the same at the end as the start. It's a powerful combination, leaving only a little room for simply recording or commenting on day to day events. We determine to be honest about our past and present choices, thoughts and actions, reflecting on these to understand how they have limited us or are limiting our future.

We also need to somehow keep reconnecting to what really matters to us, because that changes as we change, as we journey from where we are now to living the life we really want to live.

When we journal, we find that we connect to our inner wisdom and longings again, opening our heart and mind to possibilities, and then helping us examine

5

those in the light of all our experience, and make wiser choice about what happens next.

ANCIENT JOURNALS

As a practice, we know that journaling goes back for thousands of years, as the evidence is there in clay tablets, papyrus, Pergamum and paper. It's a practice found around the world and in different (and no) faiths. In the second century A.D., Marcus Aurelius wrote his "Meditations" (now available freely on the internet), recording his private spiritual reflections on his Stoic beliefs, on trying to be a "good man," and his time as a Roman Emperor.

It is believed he just wrote it for himself, but much of what he wrote is helpful for us now, such as his thinking on not catastrophizing what is happening in our lives right now, and remembering how resilient we really are:

"Do not assemble in your mind the many and varied troubles which have come to you in the past and will come again in the future, but ask yourself with regard to every present difficulty: "What is there in this that is unbearable and beyond endurance?"

St Augustine's "Confessions," written in the fourth century is both a memoir and a journal, capturing his life, his spiritual journey, and his efforts to discipline his mind and practice. He often used guided questions

6

to formalize his thinking and beliefs, simply writing down his own question and then writing out his answer.

In the 10th century, wealthy Japanese women used journals to record significant events and write a form of poetry called Waku, or they recorded poetry or dreams in the "pillowbooks" that were kept in the bedroom. By Victorian times, keeping a journal was a common practice, at a time when there were strict moral codes to be observed externally and there may well have been an element of therapy involved in their writing. Queen Victoria kept extensive journals. Perhaps this was a very useful release when there were few she could unburden herself to or make unrestricted comments to. The interest in journals and diaries was maintained through the early part of the 20th Century, and there are many war diaries that make fascinating historical and personal records.

MODERN JOURNALING

It wasn't until the mid-twentieth century though, that journaling first started to be properly examined and researched as a therapeutic tool, by Dr Ira Progof , held to be the "father" of journaling as we know it now. He was curious about how people could live a fulfilling life, and he knew that journaling was popular with certain groups of people.

He also believed that everyone had inner wisdom they could tap into, to find meaning in life events. This got him thinking about using journaling as a tool to purposefully live a "fulfilling life," and over time, this led to the development of his Intensive Journal to encourage this to happen. It offered different approaches and tools including accessing meditative states to write, and recalling and logging memories in a particular way to help do that. His ongoing research found that his clients were able to process memories, thoughts and feelings in a healthier way.

Although the use of journaling as a therapeutic tool was to increase after this, it was only towards the end of the twentieth century that extensive research started to take place about the effects and impact of journaling.

While I'm here, a brief mention of bullet journaling. You may well find bullet journaling helpful; it's a specific system to gather information and organize your life, but it's not a tool for personal transformation and growth. If you like systems, this may work for you – but please try active journaling where you don't need to colour inside the lines.

2. THE SCIENTIFIC BENEFITS OF JOURNALING

By thoroughly fixing your gaze upon yourself, you must awaken to the reality of your own existence.

— BEOP JEONG

PAYING ATTENTION TO YOUR LIFE

Professor Richard J Davidson found that happiness was a skill that could be learned by paying attention to your life by a variety of contemplative practices. Journaling is a contemplative practice that helps us pay attention to our life and focus on who we want to be and what we want to do at a time when we can be distracted by so many things. Blaise Pascal said he had discovered that the habit of distraction was responsible for all the unhappiness of men. In a digital world where we find it increasingly difficult to switch off, it is little wonder that mindfulness is becoming increasingly popular – and important.

Mindfulness is the deliberate practice of being present in the moment, a useful tool for anxiety and worry that keep us in the past or put us in the future, where we tell ourselves stories (most of which never come through). But what if you want to not just stay in the present, but plan for your future and learn from your past? What if you want to awaken to the reality of your life and your existence? Then more is required.

It's important that you know what you are paying attention to, because what you pay attention to impacts all of your life, even the bits you aren't aware of consciously.

THE MIND-BODY CONNECTION

Let's look at this in more detail. Your mind – how you think, your conscious thoughts and your unconscious thoughts – affect your body, effecting physical changes and feelings. When you think about any particular thing or experience, your feelings will range somewhere on a continuum from highly positive to highly negative. If the thing you are thinking about is related to a phobia or fear, or a deep and lasting memory,

then some of your subsequent behaviours and feelings, are instinctive and immediate (and not always
helpful).

Just stop and see how strong this automatic reac-
tion is by choosing a particular memory to focus on,
or by thinking about a person you really disliked,
something you've a phobia of, a time when you were
really happy or sad, or that time you were at the other
end of road rage and it wasn't funny. What feelings
come up? What other memories does it trigger? Do
you feel you had any power over your thoughts, feelings or any action? You probably didn't feel that
you had.

It's not just our driving that is often done without
thinking; much of our lives are on autopilot. We do
many things without really knowing how or why we
do them, or why we continue to do them. We've just
always done them, or done them for so long that they
feel like part of us, and it's only when someone
queries what is happening that we start thinking more
deeply about it, and start questioning ourselves. In the
absence of anyone querying our behaviours, actions
or thinking, how could we start to ask questions of
ourselves, or find answers? For when we start to notice
all the stuff we aren't really paying attention to, or
these unconscious thoughts that could be highly valu-
able to notice, or change, we soon surprise ourselves.

CONSCIOUSLY CREATING YOUR LIFE

The scientific research shows journaling supports you to pay attention to your life, to slow yourself down enough to notice what is happening. It allows you to transfer your thinking on to paper, and that's where emotions like fear/anger/resentment/pain lose much of their power when written down in black and white. In black and white, you can investigate them properly, examining the evidence for and against. If you aren't a ruminator and are not dealing with trauma, it can help you deal with emotions gently. It helps you to deal with old memories in a safe place with no judgement, allow you to notice patterns and beliefs you weren't aware of, and helps you remember details you are no longer consciously aware of.

It can also help you notice how you feel physically when writing certain things. It can help you plan and achieve goals by breaking bigger tasks down. It can help you change the language you use so it helps you be stronger or more resilient, and it can help you change the stories you tell yourself, by starting to rewrite them so you allow yourself to notice the negative and pain, or how you keep distracting yourself so you can ignore the negative and pain. It can help you see what might be triggering certain moods or responses AND help you change the feelings connected with them.

It allows you to know that even if you allow your-self to sit with a feeling that it DOES pass – and you don't die. It gives you a place to go when you need time to reflect or breathe that's always available and non-judgemental. If you review what you've written and reflect on it, you can make changes using the information and insight you've gained *with hindsight* to see how you can make improvements to your life now, or how you would handle things differently. So if you are suffering from stress, for instance, by recording what makes your stress worse or how it makes you feel, that can be really helpful information to share with a manager or a GP or counsellor.

IMPROVE YOUR MENTAL AND PHYSICAL HEALTH

The great news is that there's no particular group of people or type of individual that journaling works for (Christensen et al (1996). Social factors, background, age, demographics, sex, intelligence are all irrelevant. It just works – and here are some of the reasons why it's not just good for your mental health: it's good for your physical health too.

Stephen Lapore of Carnegie Mellon University showed that students who wrote about their emotions suffered fewer symptoms of mental distress. This was confirmed by studies by Greenberg et al (1996),

Smyth (1998), Spera et al (1994), Pennebaker and Francis (1996) who said those who journal are less depressed and have a better overall mood. Paez et all (1999)) said journaling led to a better day mood and Kovac and Range (2002) found it reduced suicidal thoughts.

Klein & Boals (2001) and later, Sloan & Marx (2004) said it helped with Post Traumatic Stress Disorder (PTSD), helping people reduce nightmares and the unexpected flashbacks of traumatic events while helping them reconnect to places and activities they had been avoiding. This is of course best done with the support of professionals who deal in trauma.

Its benefits have been shown in people who are grieving, who have lived with alcoholic parents or a child with a chronic illness, for those going through relationship breakups (or potential break ups). It reduces the impact of OCD and obsessive thinking.

Even where you weren't directly writing about a *particular* problem, the research found that people who wrote benefitted from expressing themselves and emotionally processing things, when they wrote the way they wanted to for as little as 20 minutes at a time three or four times on consecutive days or weeks. (Smyth & Pennebaker, 1999). A few years later, Farb et al (2010) concluded that it was the focus on the

14

emotions and feelings that made the difference, by allowing these to be processed rather than avoiding or ignoring. It is, after all, a powerful thing to sit with an emotion, and learn that it will not destroy you.

Research shows it also improves your body and physical health and wellbeing. Your immune system benefits (as long as you are processing emotions effectively), your blood pressure lowers, there are short term changes in your heart rate, and chronic illnesses are improved (as are liver and lung functions).

In fact your whole life benefits – it improves student's grades, working memory, sporting performance, even your chances of being re-employed after being made redundant. That it works to improve your physical, mental and emotional wellbeing is now undisputed – so let's get practical by delving deeper into why it matters that *you* journal.

3. WHY IT MATTERS THAT YOU JOURNAL

Only when we are brave enough to explore our darkness will we discover the infinite power of our light.

— BRENE BROWN

YOUR REALITY IS CREATED FROM WHAT YOU THINK, FEEL AND DO

Change your thinking, you change your life has been said by so many different thought leaders. It's that simple – and that hard, because up to now you may not have understood the power your thinking has on your life, or believed that you could change or manage what you thought. You might not be aware of limiting beliefs or outdated values that are running your life for you - but by regularly observing your life, you'll get to see these and then you can do something to change them so they work for you. It's often not the actual thought that ultimately matters; it's what you attach to that thought that counts, for that also affects your body, emotions, moods and actions. Think about it – everyone can change in an instant from being happy to angry, sad or fearful just be <u>one</u> thought, even though they were perfectly fine before it. Think of what happens if you get bad news, if someone says something upsetting to you, if a particular memory comes up.

Learning to change your thoughts changes your life. You will start to see that much of what you believe is not a statement of immovable fact once you start examining your beliefs. Whose belief is it? Do you still really believe this to be true? Are you relying on fake facts? Can you find clear evidence to contradict even your firmly held belief (remembering that we usually hone in and focus on evidence that support our beliefs)?

The Guardian newspaper did an interesting experiment with individuals' in the US 2016 Election, asking them to follow different sites and people on their Facebook pages than what they would normally do, in the last month of the election. Check it out to see how uncomfortable most people found it to be.

It matters what you watch and listen to, and how

18

you spend your time. It matters that you pay attention to your life, because life is not a dress rehearsal, and our lives are often lived so mindlessly - even when we know we want to be happier, healthier, kinder, richer, or wiser - and we often know what it would take to live like that. When we don't know what is stopping us live the way we want, we need to find those answers . It matters that you journal.

When you journal, you start dealing with your emotions, to process painful emotions healthily so they don't make you ill. You also learn to access the emotions you've been running away or hiding from, and feel them. You will learn to live with them and even master these.

You will learn to identify and change the beliefs that have limited your life to date, including those that your inner critic swears are true. Remember that it's your mind's job to be right and it's your inner critic's job to protect you. It does this by negative comments and beliefs –but just because you hear this voice in your head doesn't mean you have to listen to it, or that anything it says is actually true.

You learn to probe memories frozen in time, and deal with them from a mature and healthier place. You learn to be gentler on yourself as you understand yourself more, and even rewrite your story.

DARE TO BE HAPPIER

You will dare to be happier. Fordyce (1977) concluded that there are fourteen fundamental things that contribute to our own happiness. Of these, journaling helps us in nearly every area, from getting better organised and planning things out, to stopping worrying, lowering our expectations and aspirations and develop positive, optimistic thinking. It helps us be ourselves, become present-oriented, work on having a healthier personality, eliminate negative feelings and problems and improve our relationships. It also helps us put happiness as our most important priority, so you find out what makes you happy and how to get there. You reconnect with your heart; a vital tool for happiness.

> *Many of the great sorrows of the world arise when the mind is disconnected to the heart.*

— JACK KORNFIELD

In her book The How of Happiness: A Scientific Approach to Getting the Life You Want, Sonja Lyubomirsky argues that 50% of happiness is determined by genetics, 10% by life circumstances, and 40% by our habits, values, behaviours and thinking.

Journaling will help maximise this 40% you DO have control of, by giving you a space to do what she suggests, by practicing gratitude and positive thinking (expressing gratitude, cultivating optimism and avoiding overthinking), by improving social connections, by managing stress, hardship or trauma by developing coping strategies and learning to forgive) and by living in the present.

To live in the present moment means we must face what is - and that's why journaling is so powerful. We can no longer avoid ourselves. We truly meet ourselves here, even those parts of us that we deny or avoid, with love and in peace. It creates a safe space for me to be present. I am in the cocoon, quietly transforming, finding my questions and answering them, being reminded of my inner wisdom, worth and beauty. Then, I learn to resolve my anxiety and worries, and in the darkness, get the strength to dream of and create a better future. I stretch my wings. I fly. I discover the infinite power of my life.

The world outside you doesn't transform until you transform yourself.

— CESAR MILAN

A journal is also a tool for self-discovery, an aid to concentration, a mirror for the soul, a place to generate and capture ideas, a safety valve for the emotions, a training ground for the writer, and a good friend and confidant.

— RON KLUG

4. HOW TO JOURNAL

I hate rules, and the older I get the less likely I am to conform to rules anyway. There are very few "rules" about journaling, so you really don't need to worry about "getting it right."

Here are the top five journaling rules that are best followed:

1. Anyone who is severely depressed, suffers from high levels of anxiety, has Post Traumatic Stress Disorder, has unresolved trauma in their life or ruminates (thinks circularly or passively about an issue) is unlikely to benefit without the addition of expert help to support you – so seek that out.

2. Where possible, use pen and paper, as that allows your creativity to flow.

3. You must write only for yourself. It doesn't matter about grammar, punctuation, legibility. Since honesty (no holds barred, no judgement or censoring) is vital, you will need to ensure that you can write freely and privately. If this cannot be assured, you *can* now journal by using your computer, either through password protected documents or through a variety of software options. Or you can write on scrap paper and then burn it or shred it immediately afterwards. Don't run from your own story; allow yourself the privilege of getting to know yourself – darkness and light. Reconnect with your heart, inspire, nurture and encourage yourself – and be willing to observe your present life as it is. Be willing to explore your past and future, your emotions (great happiness as well as despair), your dreams and plans and goals, and to access your own inner wisdom. Above all, be gentle on yourself.

4. Make time to journal: if you are too busy to journal, you are too busy. You have time to do everything else you are doing. Let go

of one of them to make the time for this, even if it means letting go of 20 minutes sleep; the changes you see will be worth that investment in your own inner life. Starting small is all that matters.

5. There are no other rules.

Here are some things that aren't rules, but help:

Though any notebook or paper will do just fine, choosing to use a lovely journal can be seen as a way of nurturing yourself. Some people personalise their journals, some use the cheapest journals they can find, while others prefer to use blank paper, as they feel more freedom to deviate from lines and add pictures, charts etc. I personally find that writing in a lovely journal helps my mind work better, but I've scribbled on all sorts of paper, including napkins and receipts.

Rituals can help in setting and maintaining this as a spiritual practice, whether that is sitting in the same chair at the same time each morning, listening to a particular piece of music, meditating beforehand, or lighting a candle while you journal.

You can journal on a daily, weekly or monthly basis, although you will benefit most when you do it regularly, and commit to a schedule where you do it even when you are not in the mood. Skipping days is a normal part of journaling. No-one is forcing you to do anything and you don't have to listen to that voice that says "oh no, I should be journaling". Unless of course, you should! The more you commit to it, the more you will get from it.

You can use pencils or pens, you can always use the same colour of pen, have different colours of pens for different people, or events, or feelings, to highlight them (as long as you remember your "code"). Use diagrams, doodles, drawings. Stick, paint, cut out and fold over to your heart's content. It's entirely up to you.

5. WHAT DO I WRITE ?

This is probably the question asked most often by those who have never tried any type of journaling before. The journal is opened - and panic rises, as all sorts of memories of being asked to do creative writing at school rear their head - and limiting beliefs emerge, and mental barriers shoot up.

These barriers are what we use every time we are encouraged to experiment, but fear failure. One of our greatest lessons is that whatever we do in life, there is no failure; only feedback about how we can do things differently next time. When we are learning a new skill, competence isn't expected - and nor is perfection. Relax. Be curious about what you might find out about yourself and your thinking (including your need to be in control, or perfect).

Remember that you aren't at school. No one is

going to mark or judge your writing skills, grammar or punctuation. None of that matters because you aren't writing an essay or thesis. "Write as you would if you were writing to someone you know," I will say. "Just write." It doesn't have to be War and Peace; it can be a sentence or two.

If you are really stuck, take time to find a question about your life that you really want to figure the answer out for, and have the courage to sit with that question, turning it over in your head until some thoughts about it start to emerge. We all have these thoughts running through our head; journaling captures these and allows you to examine them, challenge them, deal with them or let them go.

Write those down, and see what happens next. There's no pressure. There's no need for pressure, as this is about your own personal development, so being gentle on yourself is a good start. As you become more conscious of how you are living your life, and as you want to improve it, you will soon find inspiration everywhere!

Let's give an example of a day in the life of Maria, who's turned up for her first evening at an introduction to journaling course. She sits down on her chair, finds her journal and a pen, and her thoughts go something like this.

Whew. I made it, even though the traffic was a nightmare

and I left a bit late as I was trying to catch up on all the housework before I came. I'm such a poor time manager! But at least now I can sit down and relax a bit I hope. What a day I've had, today, sleeping in like that. It wasn't enough to make me late for work, just enough to mean that my normal routine was shot to pieces. My day didn't get better. I spilt coffee over my desk, an important meeting I was supposed to have got cancelled, I'm struggling with a project deadline, and my partner didn't pick up his phone to arrange emergency childcare cover, so I ended up having to ask to leave work a bit early.

I worked through lunch, and as I came straight to the course, I haven't had time for dinner, just grabbing a coffee and a chocolate bar, so now I'm feeling really tired. I really want to find out about journaling, but I'm spinning so many plates this weather that I'm dizzy. I'm always chasing my tail. There's never enough time in the day for everything I want to do. I'll sit here and listen, but I'm actually pretty upset. I've no idea why I even turned up, really, as I can't write for tuppence. I'm so useless at life!

As Maria sits with her journal, reflecting, she might start to see some of her beliefs about herself and capture those (like "I'm such a poor time manager," "I'm so useless at life," and "I can't write for tuppence.") She could think about her day. What went wrong with her alarm? What happened today that

29

was less than totally positive? What would she want to do differently tomorrow?

Is there a particular relationship or conversation on her mind? Where did she feel stuck today? She is feeling upset, and anxious - why might that be? What else is she worried or anxious about? What decisions did she make today and was she happy with her choices? How can she get that project back on track? As she is feeling stressed, and out of balance, is it time to do something about that, or her time management skills? What might that be? What can she delegate? Where does she need to put better boundaries in place? Who could she ask for help? What could she just stop doing? What is she avoiding?

These are just some of the things that her thoughts might bring up that could do with further exploration. She could write some of these thought down and think carefully about them, or just write out how she is feeling, or she could at least note them, so she can do that later on. If she wants to change her mood, she could try changing her focus so she no longer feels so unhappy and upset. That would put her in a better frame of mind for learning. That would mean different questions of course. The questions we ask ourselves are the most important ones for our growth. Be curious.

Now, she could ask:

Where did I find beauty, happiness or kindness

today? What did I think about doing differently today, and what am I going to do next about that? What can I be grateful for? What is good in this present moment? If I'm retelling the story of this day in a month's time, where would I find humour?

Even just one attempt to journal can change your life, if you're relaxed, open and curious. Baby steps still get you to the top of any hill or mountain. Simply reflecting on how one day has gone will be enough to open up lots to explore further. That's enough to get anyone started. In the next section, I share the seven best journaling tools to help you know "what else to write."

6. REVIEWING YOUR JOURNALS

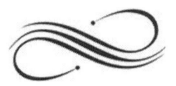

Some people choose to never review their journals. That means that either they end up being piled up in boxes in attics, or they get thrown out in a decluttering mood or a house move. Perhaps you are the kind of person who isn't interested in the past and just want to keep moving forward. Or perhaps it's because there is so much pain captured in the journals that you don't want to revisit that, or else reviewing them makes you feel a failure as you see how often you write about similar things, or notice you still haven't got very far with what you once promised yourself to do. That means that if you ever DO choose to re-read your journals, it's imperative that you do so in a spirit of curiosity and gentleness towards yourself.

If rereading them would remind you mainly of pain, if the thought of them weighs heavily on you, or if you definitely wouldn't want someone else reading them, then sometimes it is wiser to let them go. If you decide to do that, create a ritual to let what you've written go. Light a fire, light candles. Pour a glass of wine and put uplifting music on. Use an open fire or one built for a barbeque, or find a way to light one. Bless what you've written, honour your commitment to your growth, and ask that any wisdom that is needed from it will stay with you. Tear the pages up into pieces and set fire to them, and watch as they curl up and the smoke ascends to the sky. When I did this, I found it hugely cathartic – and the patterns left on crisped paper to be fascinating and beautiful.

AN ONGOING PROCESS

Otherwise, reviewing journals is part of the magic. You can zone in on a particular period of time, or re-read it all. Make re-reading your journals an ongoing process. It's the best way to see what keeps cropping up in your life, habits like procrastination, or not taking action and what you're afraid of. Klug (2002) calls this harvesting our journals, bringing back all the good things and treasure with you, like lessons learned, patterns recognised, goals reached, things to be grateful for.

Sometimes you will look back and laugh at what you wrote, sometimes you will be thankful that period in your life has passed, while at other times you won't even be able to remember the situation that caused you so much angst. When you are reviewing your journal, read it with compassion or curiosity, as a loving, kind friend would read it.

I always review one journal before moving on to the next, pulling out any wisdom (words to live by, patterns, goals not yet achieved, questions), and move them to the front pages of my new journal. I use that to set the intention for the journal I'm about to start. I also review them half way through the year, and at the end of the year to see what I need to focus on for the year ahead. After that, I don't tend to keep my journals now.

The review at the end of the year doesn't lead to me making resolutions, though it may do to that for you. Since 2005, it has led to a major theme I recognise I need or want to develop in my life. That's led me to have adventures in love and new beginnings, developing an attitude of gratitude, moving from debt to grace, learning to say yes – and no, finding my voice, finding balance, seeing miracles, building connections that matter, letting go, being awesome and being still and learning patience.

Experiment; find out what works for you. If you remove the writing you don't want, it may even inspire you to use what's left to create works of art that include your words torn into shapes or cut out, with painting and other media or craft materials. Use your journal and the reviewing process to connect again to your heart. You will have found you can listen carefully to your soul and inner wisdom, even at times when other people's voices - or your own fears - are drowning that out. And you will have realised you have the courage to do this self-exploration, to stare yourself in the face and see your darkness and your light and accept who you are - and all your possibilities.

II

THE SEVEN BEST
JOURNALING TOOLS

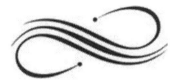

1. FREESTYLE JOURNALING

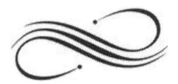

If you aren't a regular writer, and aren't used to expressing your thoughts or emotions, the thought of just sitting down to write can seem daunting. All sorts of fears crowd in, so your inner critic has you putting up barriers like:

What if it brings up memories or feelings I don't like? *These memories are always better out than in; they still need processed. Learn to sit with your emotions in a safe place.*

I can't possibly share my deepest darkest thoughts! *Yet you are darkness and light. Running from such thoughts or ignoring them doesn't mean they don't exist. Let them be seen. Learn to drop shame. Process and reframe them, you wonderfully imperfect human being.*

I don't let go. I hold everything in. *Learn to let go to move forward.*

I couldn't trust what comes up if I write, so why bother? *If you've not listened to it for a while, there could be a reluctance to trust your inner wisdom; that will come with practice.*

Our fears that we might fail, or not get things "right" may initially stop us – but freewriting is such a wonderful tool because there *is* no right or wrong – therefore no chance of failure! It was a creative process used by writers to stop writers block and just get in the mood for writing; the very practice of picking up a pen and starting to write can be enough to do this. 10 or 15 minutes is enough.

Just open your journal and start writing, with no agenda, word limit or decisions about what to write about. Your head will be full of thoughts, so just grab one and start writing, or write about yesterday, your plans for the day, an event, memory, person or question that's on your mind. Just write out what comes up, without filtering or correcting anything.

Your mind might initially resist, but by persevering, you break through that resistance. It's likely your writing will jump from thought to thought, that much of it won't make sense, or that things you didn't

40

expect will pop into your head. When you review what you've written (some say to do this by reading out loud), it may well fail to generate much of note – but what it *does* generate will be worth the effort.

You will slowly begin to uncover memories, beliefs and feelings that lie dormant but need addressed – things that are causing you stress, making you sabotage yourself, or hold you back in relationships or careers. You may come up with solutions to problems that have bothered you for a while. You will remember and reconnect with dreams and hopes, and find ways to overcome your fears in achieving them. This tool alone may help you find the courage to live the life you really want.

2. GUIDED JOURNALING

Journaling is a reflective tool and one of the best ways to reflect is by answering questions. We don't all have people who we can talk to, or people who are brave enough to ask us the right questions, so that is where guided journaling can be helpful.

Sometimes, one question is all that is needed to have a breakthrough. At other times, it is helpful to have a series of questions that take us deeper into a particular theme, as the best diamonds are always in the deepest mines. That process will often start off lightly, to get us started, take us deeper via a series of structured questions, and then take us back up with questions that move us forward. It's just you exploring your own thinking.

It can be a really useful tool, prompting further study or action.

You will find yourself adding notes, doodles, stars, carry things forward to the back of your journal or a different journal to plan, take action or remember (like a gratitude journal).

You can ask yourself questions as you go along, ask a series of questions, or use prompts like the following:

How did I look after my physical (mental or spiritual) wellbeing today?

What did I learn from how I handled something today?

What thoughts did I exaggerate today?

What evidence do I have that this thought was true? Wasn't true?

What would a kind and compassionate loving friend say to me just now?

What can I be grateful for today?

Where did I manage to be present in the moment today?

What did I give to others today?

How was I kind to others today?

How was I kind to myself today?

What strategies have I found helpful in the past?

What strategies did I use to help myself today?

What is the one thing I need most in the world right now?

What feelings did I make room for today?

How did I stretch my comfort zones today?

How much is my expectation of perfection impacting my ability to live a life I love?

Or choose one word and then see where you would have done things differently e.g. example, educate, inspire, love, improve, help, be patient with, motivate, nurture, understand etc.

3. REFLECTIVE JOURNALING

This is where you take time to deliberately reflect on a previous day, or a situation at work or socially to learn any lessons from it. It's good for leaders to use, or anyone interested in personal development. You write out what happened, how you felt, or what you will do differently next time. It is a useful tool to keep learning, stops certain behaviours becoming an ongoing issue - and stops you continually thinking about it.

Benjamin Franklin had a Virtue Journal which he used to help him live a better life. He chose 13 "virtues" to focus on for 13 week periods at a time, which meant he concentrated on each group four times each year. Each evening, he would reflect on how well the thought he had lived in line with each virtue, carefully noting his progress on his temperance (vs overindulgence), silence (or really only speaking when he had something of importance to say), order, resolution (keeping his promises to himself and others), frugality (waste nothing), industry (hard work and making a good use of time), sincerity, justice, moderation (by avoiding extremes), cleanliness, tranquility, chastity and humility (added to the original list of 12 because a friend advised him he was considered to be too proud).

He created a book, which had a page for each week, seven columns for each day of the week and 13 rows for the weeks. He would concentrate on one virtue for a whole week at a time (a wise move, as smaller steps are always easier than trying to accomplish a lot at the same time).

Where he felt he hadn't lived up to a virtue, he would add a black spot, and then concentrate on not having a spot for the next day. Initially he had many black spots, but this concentration and reflection led to him changing his behavior and habits, and though he had (unreasonably) aimed at perfection, he was able to conclude that he was, *"by the endeavour, a better and a happier man than I otherwise should have been if I had not attempted it."*

Another option is to ask the questions suggested by Alcoholics Anonymous in Chapter 6 of their "Big Book," which are:

- Were we resentful, selfish, dishonest or afraid?
- Do we owe an apology?
- Have we kept something to ourselves which should be discussed with another person at once? Were we kind and loving toward all?
- What could we have done better?
- Were we thinking of ourselves most of the time?
- Or were we thinking of what we could do for others, of what we could pack into the "stream of life?"

Or you may just decide to reflect on the same question each night, such as "Was I true to myself today?" or "Did I nurture myself today", or "How did I nurture myself today," or "What could I have done differently today," or "What am I proud of today?"

4. PROPRIOCEPTIVE WRITING

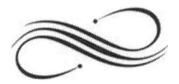

This technique was developed by Linda Trichter Metcalf and Tobin Simon. It means that you free write for a continuous period of set time, but as you write, you are encouraged to note things that attract your conscious attention. Normally, you would keep writing a longer "stream of thinking," and wait to the end to review it. Here, you notice what attracts your attention, and then you follow that thought wherever it goes, specifically questioning what it brings up. It is a means of getting to know who you are, even the parts that may be "blind" to you.

Like all journaling, there is the ritual of pen and paper, though here you must only use plain paper so there are no restrictions. There is freedom to write how and where you want to, and freedom to draw and doodle (as you are encouraged to keep your pen moving all the time as in stream of consciousness writing). As there are no lines to stay inside, you can even break your own rules.

You start by lighting a candle and by playing baroque music because that induces alpha waves in your brain, calming you down and producing a state of "relaxed awareness" that is considered key to concentration.

You set a timer for a defined period of 20-25 minutes, start writing, starting with the first thought in your mind, if you haven't a specific idea you want to explore (possibly from a previous "Write." Keep writing, without judgement - but as you are writing mindfully, you will begin to notice what you are writing and the words you are using. A particular word will catch your attention, you will see you've spelt something differently (e.g. write where you meant right), or an idea or memory will seem to pop into your mind from nowhere.

These are the key pivot points; points of transition, where you deliberately ask yourself a question about what you have noticed. The easiest option is to always ask "What do I mean by?" e.g. "What do I mean by ....spelling that word like that?" or "What do I mean by..... sadness?" or "What do I mean by... had enough now?" You will find yourself changing direction many times – and finding many insights.

When the timer goes, you ask four final questions, which are important parts of the process:

1. What thoughts were heard but not written?
2. How or what do I feel now?
3. What larger story is the Write part of?
4. What ideas came up for future Writes

5. WRITING FROM A DIFFERENT ANGLE

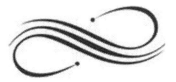

We are all individuals with different backgrounds, abilities, experiences, beliefs etc., these affect how we behave in life - and we're not always right and nor is the other person. Conflict and difficulties in relationships arise for a number of reasons, but it often comes down either to misunderstanding what happened, or by making assumptions about why something was said or done. We are told not to judge anyone until we have walked a mile in their moccasins. It's good advice.

It might not even be an issue of right or wrong, just of these differences, and then allowing ourselves to get entrenched by our hurt in our view of our own wisdom. In the trenches, we dig ourselves deeper and deeper, and become afraid to put our head above the parapet to wave any kind of white flag. When both parties do this, war can be declared. Often you will read of people who no longer talk, of family feuds where no-one remembers what started it all. Life is too short for that sort of anger and hurt in your life.

Where you genuinely want to find a way forward, and want to try to understand what's happened, trying to see things from a different point of view can help shift things, even without directly speaking to them – and even if they are dead.

When you commit to this, you can write a break-through. You may not be correct in *any* of your conclusions about their thinking, feelings or behaviours, but really that doesn't matter. It's your openness to learning to see something differently that matters.

It's a technique you can do yourself that is similar to those you might use with a counsellor using Gestalt's Empty Chair Technique or NLP's Perceptual Positions. You agree to willingly put yourself in the other person's position while being open to the fact that you may not be wholly or even partially "right." You will write about the situation(s) or event(s) that led to the impasse from that person's perspective; you will tell *their* story. Use your imagination and see where it can take you. As you go along, "notice" what they might be thinking, questions or observations they might have, as well as what they say and how they say it. It is okay to note briefly (in the margin) anything you are feeling and thinking yourself as you try to see from a different point of view. If it helps, because you're worried it may be deeply hurtful, imagine yourself doing this through the closed window of a house, as that will give you a protective screen to start looking at it.

It's also really helpful to do this from the view of an objective third party, and see what comes up, or from your future self, or from your higher self (where you want only the best, and believe that all you experience is ultimately good). Or to do from a point in the future, where you write a letter to your future self, about what you had learned or done.

At the end of the exercise, review what you've written. Ask what they are teaching you, or hoping to teach you, or write about what you noticed about how you felt at different points.

6. GRATITUDE JOURNALING

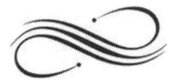

Gratitude journaling is simply listing three or five things each day you are really grateful for. This more than anything will help you to stay positive. You take control of your emotions, which are always your responsibility. You don't have to be controlled by them though it is good to be guided by them (and feel them or take action as a result of them). This then makes you take control of your own happiness level, as you practice finding silver linings, reasons to be cheerful.

There's lots of scientific evidence to support this. It started being researched on the back of the positive psychology movement resulting from Maslow and Seligman's studies on what kept people mentally healthy as opposed to focussing on trying to fix people once that had started to deteriorate. In 1998, Dr Emmons was going to be attending a conference that

looked at different virtues (forgiveness, humility, gratitude); he was asked to become a gratitude expert and
talk about it for an hour. His research (along with
McCullough) showed him how powerful this one
virtue was, as the reality was that it – along with hope,
optimism and happiness - didn't depend on circumstances or genetics.

By practising gratitude, people reported feeling
better, sleeping better, being more optimistic, making
better connections and feeling less pain. In organisations, employees felt better connected to where they
worked if employers were grateful for their contribu-
tion. Bartlett and McCullough's research found
similar conclusions, with increased exercise levels,
enthusiasm, energy, determination to achieve goals, as
well as increased levels of interest in and emotional
support for others. Froh, Sefick, & Emmons, (2008)
reported that children who practice gratitude have
more positive attitudes toward school and their
families.

I know it works. 2006 was an annus horribilus for
me. I forgot all I knew, stopped journaling, went from
being someone who normally excelled at whatever she
did to doubting my ability to do anything well. I had
severe symptoms of stress and ended up taking three
months off work, and when I did work, I came home,
got into my pyjamas, curled up and shut out the
world, becoming increasingly depressed. It was a dark

time. Then someone asked me what I was grateful for. I looked blankly at them. They said to get back to journaling, and start with a gratitude journal, finding three things each day to be grateful for, as this would start to take my focus off all that wasn't working. When your mind is solely focussed only on what isn't working, that's less than easy to do.

Later, when I got into bed, I pulled out a journal and sat in tears, trying to think of one thing I was grateful for. It took me one hour to think of one thing, and that was my electric blanket. Something easy to take for granted, but without which I struggled to sleep. Two hours later, I had my three things, the third being a hot cup of tea that my husband brought to me. It was the start of my adventures in gratitude (and it showed me that anything we do can be hard work and start very small, but is often worth persevering with). It changed my life – and *now* I could write pages of what I'm grateful for.

7. CLUSTERING

When you are stuck or things don't seem to be making any sense, it can be helpful to use a quick tool that unsticks our thinking. When we stop to observe our thoughts, we soon realise how much they jump about from subject to random subject. Yet there may be real nuggets of wisdom in there, if we could capture the thinking OR unlock our thinking, particularly if it is on a particular subject.

Brainstorming attempts to capture what can seem to be random ideas that come up when people start thinking creatively about something. In business, the most common technique for brainstorming is to use sticky notes and then place them on a relevant point on a whiteboard. The Mind mapping concept that Tony Buzan introduced is a much more visual tool, using images, different coloured pens and single words rather than sentences, grouped together through a series of curved lines where ideas link up. As the process unfolds, and ideas and thoughts are very briefly analysed, these ideas start to form a structure that allows for further, logical investigation.

The structured element of mind maps mean that , to a degree, you analyse what you are writing, to put it in the "right" area. Clustering removes that element of analysis as you write. It was developed by Dr Gabriele Lusser Rico, and is a combination of mind mapping *and* free writing, drawing *and* writing. You start with a word in the centre that is the "issue" of concern, and then you just relax, dive in, and go with the flow. You focus on that first word and then write continuously, capturing all the other words or ideas that come into your head wherever you want on the page.

Each new idea or thought is circled, and can be linked to one or more thoughts if you wish. It's a rapid fire process, and without that need for structure, you relax more. It's important that the writing is continuous, so the writer is encouraged to keep the pen moving at all times, as it this that makes the links between thoughts and your creativity and inner wisdom. You write for five or ten minutes, and you keep going with that until you stop coming up with anything. If you get stuck, return to the centre again and see where that takes you this time. You will find that there are things there you wouldn't necessarily have associated with that central idea if you'd thought about it rationally and logically.

When you've finished, you then circle your main thoughts and link them to the original idea as well as checking where they link to other words or ideas on the page too. What do particular words mean? Do you see any patterns? Does something now make sense that didn't beforehand? Is there something that now really stands out?

At the end, you take a few minutes to summarise your experience, noting what surprised you, what you want to explore more, what memories it unsurfaced, what it made you want to do or find out more about.

III

52 QUESTIONS – 52 WEEKS
TO TRANSFORM YOUR LIFE

WEEKLY QUESTIONS

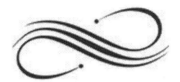

Week 1

What issues keep cropping up in your life that you know you need to address?

Week 2

What do you really need to focus on this week? How are you letting yourself be distracted?

Week 3

Where or what do you need to declutter first?

Week 4

How can you become more resilient to deal with change better?

Week 5

How are you supporting your own happiness and wellbeing?

Week 6

If you can't change your circumstances, what thoughts could you start to change about them?

Week 7

What have you learned from your failures? What mistakes are you grateful for?

Week 8

Think back to a story that you use to define yourself in a less than totally positive way. What if you viewed this from a different person's angle? What elements of the story do you always leave out? How could you reframe the story to help you move forward?

Week 9

Endings are beginnings. What do any new beginnings you are facing mean to you? How can you honour the endings and embrace the beginnings?

Week 10

What are you worrying about? What options do you have? Find one solution for each worry. If you can't see options, who do you I know is good at generating options?

Week 11

How and where do you keep the peace rather than rocking the boat?

Week 12

How do you define a great friendship? Do your current friendships support you in the way you want? What needs to change?

Week 13

What are you tolerating in your life that is not helping you?

Week 14

How do you define a great romantic relationship? How do you demonstrate love in that relationship – and what do you need them to do to demonstrate they love you? What does your romantic relationship need more of – or what's missing that used to be there?

Week 15
What are the key beliefs and words you live your
life by?

Week 16
What do you want your life to look like in one year?
In five years?

Week 17
What specifically do you still need to forgive others
for? How can you forgive yourself and move forward?

Week 18
What or who would you miss, if you no longer had it
or them in your life? Why? Do they know this?

Week 19
How do you define yourself using thoughts and
behaviours from the past that no longer support you
or are no longer relevant?

Week 20
What has your intuition/gut/inner wisdom been
trying to tell you lately? Why are you not listening?
What's your next step?

Week 21

Where are you resisting change in your life? What fears are stopping you going with the flow?

Week 22

If a loving and supportive friend was in your shoes right now, what advice would you be giving them?

Week 23

Make a list of ten things that you could do differently that would change your future?

Week 24

How do you regularly waste time? What else could you be doing that you say you don't have time for?

Week 25

How can you turn your current challenges into opportunities?

Week 26

Who and what is draining your time and energy?

Week 27

What might happen if you really connected to your heart?

Week 28

If you were to sit down and chat with someone you trusted, what would your deepest dreams be?

Week 29

In the previous week, have you spent your energy and time on the things that matter most in your life? What are your priorities and how are you organising your life around those – or what changes do you need to make to ensure you do that?

Week 30

What do you waste money on that you could use to do what you really want to do instead?

Week 31

Whose feelings are you sparing by changing who you are? Whose feelings are you sparing by staying as you are?

Week 32

What does your "ideal" week look like?

Week 33

List 30 strengths you have that you enjoy using or have enjoyed in the past. Which ones are you not using now or often, and how can you use more of them?

Week 34
What are your top 10 goals in life? How can you break those down into smaller goals to make sure you achieve them?

Week 35
How do you nurture yourself? Make yourself feel better? What things do you love to do because they inspire you or revive you?

Week 36
What excuses keep you stuck where you are?

Week 37
If your family wrote an epitaph today, what would they write? What would you LIKE them to write?

Week 38
What hidden or "lost" parts of you would you like to re-awaken?

Week 39
What do you want from your life? How are you organising your daily life around this?

Week 40
What's the difference between living your life and living a life you love, where you feel truly alive?

Week 41
What do you feel are important values in your own life and how do you know when they are being honoured? How will you live those this week?

Week 42
As you reflect on your life, what would you have done differently? What would you change? What opportunities would you have taken? What can you still do? What are you glad you did do?

Week 43
Since kindness is good for you, where will you be kinder this week (to yourself and others)? What do you learn from organised and random acts of kindness?

Week 44
What advice would you give yourself at this time in your life? (fill at least one page)

Week 45

What elements of your life would you like to see change happen in over the next year? How exactly do you want these to be different?

Week 46

Where is your life out of balance?

Week 47

What would your dream job be? What does it look like, sound like, feel like?

Week 48

Make a list of people you admire (in personal life or through the media or books). What is it that draws you to them?

Week 49

Who are the important people in your life and how are you spending the right time with them?

Week 50

What do you uniquely bring to the world? What's your purpose? How are you helping others? What are you passionate about?

Week 51

What changes in attitude and action are you committed to for the improvement of your quality of life?

Week 52

If you were taking 100 per cent care of yourself, what would you be doing differently in your life that you are not doing currently?

ABOUT THE AUTHOR

Caroline Johnstone is originally from Northern Ireland, now happily remarried and living in Ayrshire. She works part time as an Employment Law Advisor, and the rest of her time is spent running workshops where she dares people to be happier. Journaling is at the heart of every course, after she found the power of this in changing her thinking and life after her first marriage ended. After coaching informally for a number of years, she decided to train in NLP and is now a Master Practitioner and uses this – and journaling - in her coaching practice and writing.

She's also a poet, having been published in the UK, Ireland and the U.S.. She is currently a Scottish Poetry Library Ambassador, a member of the Scottish Writer's Centre and helps with the social media for the Federation of Writers (Scotland) and the cross community group Women Aloud NI.

manual for Heatache
Cathie Reatzenbrinle

Printed in Poland
by Amazon Fulfillment
Poland Sp. z o.o., Wrocław